Quick Steps To Your Better You

Motivating Moves That Take Mere Minutes To Execute

By J Cleveland Payne

ISBN-13: 978-1534987609

ISBN-10: 1534987606

Other Books By J Cleveland Payne

Welcome To Your Monday

Welcome To More Monday

So Forty Happened

Ask Yourself This

DEDICATION

This book is dedicated to my wife, Kristina with a 'K.' She knows all the hard work that went into this book. Some of it from working on the collections of minute quick hits, some of it from comically long drawn out ordeals. She knows my struggles and works through her own struggles as well. Together, we put this together, and we will put together plenty more.

HOW TO LIVE LIKE
'YOUR MISTER MONDAY'

My name is J Cleveland Payne, but for this book--*yay marketing*--you can think of me as 'Your Mister Monday.' As Your Mister Monday, I write personal development and inspiration missives and articles, and I like to believe I'm slightly internet famous.

I don't think you should try to live like me. I know I titled this passage "How To Live Like 'Your Mister Monday," but trying to live your life the way I actually live my life would be foolish. Trying to live any life other than your own is foolish. It is great to admire others, to craft your life to emulate and model others, but you cannot move on to a better you until you come to terms with the fact that you can never *be* what others are, or have been.

You can only be you. Good or bad is irrelevant.

I self-published four physical books within two years. You can buy them in paperback and everything. It was a major accomplishment, but those four books were just rungs on the ladder to this one, and this one is meant to be another rung for the next project. If there is one thing I want you to get from this book is that the journey to a 'better you' is open ended. You can get close to scoring the winning goal, but the ultimate cosmic joke is that the goal posts are always being pushed back. The game is never over. Even when you fall behind quickly, you can retake the lead at any time, just as quickly.

I don't want you to try to live like Your Mister Monday, but Your Mister Monday wants to do what he can to teach you a few things to help you get closer to your better you, whatever that is.

Let me start by debunking the whole 'Your Mister Monday' thing. What exactly is it? I already told you--*marketing*! What does the title mean? If the key to being an expert in any field is having the gall to tell people you are an expert (and hoping they connect with your content before they realize you may only know a smidgen more about the topic than they may), then consider this book me putting that key in the ignition and starting the car now. I have been teaching, training, and writing about personal development and improvement since my late teens, and I have plenty of written words to show for it, but no 'mysteriously over-hyped and grossly over-ranked' bestselling book, yet. I suspect that designation will not come from this book either, but I will not be discouraged by that. I can only be discouraged if this book fails to add anything to your work on yourself.

Despite my best intentions, I can only offer you something that I already possess. I possess a wealth of knowledge and tips and tricks, but I do not have access to anything purposefully earthshattering. Any epiphanies you gain from this book will come from the randomness of any of these tips being something you may have never heard before, or at least not in the form presented here. All wisdom must be acquired over time, and over time, you will grow to learn that most of the good stuff is commonly rehashed and restated by different people.

Think of personal development in terms of any learned subject. No one is trying to reinvent algebra, physics, or trigonometry. Some may look to expand on it, but most just want to relay the basics of what has already been proven to the next generation of learners.

This book offers tips and tricks that you can implement quickly and easily, all based on your ability to keep up with your current habits. The pacing is up to you. The effort expended is up to you.

The path to your better you is totally up to you.

There is nothing in the presentation of this book that should be considered new to the world. But I hope you find more than a few tips to be new to you that are easy to integrate into your life.

.

IT TAKES JUST A FEW MINUTES

How much time does it take for you to perform a miracle? Mere moments! It doesn't take much time for you to initiate some quick action, start some simple gesture, or do some basic movement. And for that one act alone to change the course of a day for you or other. Maybe even leading to changing and saving a life.

Perhaps your own?

Need a few ideas on what you can do in those moments when you find you have a few fleeting minutes and want to do something a little more meaningful than just glancing at your smartphone? Of course, Your Mister Monday is here to oblige.

This book, compiled from a list of motivating moves I have collected from years of research in leadership and personal improvement, was written to fit that need. The tips presented in this book are purposely written as simple and straightforward actions you can easily perform. Choose one to try, take just a few minutes of your time and watch the possibilities of great things to come into your world.

Next time you find you have a spare few minutes, why don't you consider trying one of these ideas?

Quick Steps To Your Better You

Motivating Moves That Take Mere Minutes To Execute

1

EAT A PIECE
OF
CHOCOLATE

Take a moment and indulge in your sweet tooth. One little snack won't kill the effort you've put in so far. In fact, it will help stave off the cravings that come from denying yourself of your favorite indulgence. Just make sure it is only one little snack. Take the time and slowly enjoy the experience before you get back on the wagon.

2

GIVE OF YOURSELF FREELY

There are plenty of people and organizations that could use a little of your spare time, energy, or money to accomplish its goals, some minor, some mighty. Volunteer yourself and some of your resources to a good cause, with no expectations in return.

3

MAKE A DECISION AND CHOOSE YOUR PRIORITIES

What are your most urgent tasks? The ones that must be accomplished? What actions are keeping you from completing any of these tasks? Identify the roadblocks and procrastinators that don't allow you to get the job done, and make a decision on how to eliminate them for good.

4

GO SHOPPING WITH WITH PURPOSE

On your next shopping spree, instead of blowing all your money on more things for yourself that you know you will feel guilty for later, use that urge to splurge on buying a few items that you can easily afford and just as easily donate to charity. Get a double boost for your ego for every dollar spent by targeting brands or companies that regularly donate a portion of their earnings to charity.

5

TAKE ONE OFF THE SHELF

Most people have large stashes of books around their house or office. Stashes so large that they can never find time--and will never find the time--to read a large portion of them. But you don't have to find time to read your entire library. Just select one book and start there.

6

USE EVERY SPACE AS A PLACE

Decide what items live where in your home or your office, and put them in their place. Having dedicated space for items and dedicated space for open space will help you keep your surroundings clean and organized, with little need for frenzied clean-up sessions when you are expecting company.

7

PUT YOUR SCHEDULED CHECK-UPS ON A REAL LIST

Make a physical list of all your doctor and dentist appointments and put that list on display in plain sight for everyone in your household to see. Use the same place to display a similar listing of all your doctor's and dentist's appointments that you need to schedule, but have been putting off. Having your lists on public display will give those who care about you and need you the most the chance to keep track on whether you are doing what's important to take care of yourself.

8

WRITE DOWN THREE BIG GOALS TO FOCUS ON FOR THE NEXT THREE MONTHS

Any day is a good day to tackle a new goal. It is the act of choosing the right number of goals to work on and giving yourself the right amount of time to gauge actual progress is what creates the sense of urgency necessary to do the work to reach a goal. Only choose three goals with a short deadline of three months for some resolution. When your 90 or so days have run out on your three goals, select a new triple set of goals to focus on, and reset the clock for another 90 or so days. If you are successful in accomplishing just two out of three each quarter, you should be able to claim, with pride that you conquered eight big goals in a year's time. Most people will make a list of 10 or more resolutions every January 1st, and then usually bail out before accomplishing one.

9

REMEMBER THAT SIMPLE GESTURES CAN MEAN A LOT

Don't knock the compounding effect of a few well timed simple gestures. Reach for your spouse's hand, and don't be afraid to hold it in public. Open doors to cars or buildings. Bring home flowers on a random Tuesday. Surprise them with a 'just thinking about you' greeting card.

10

SIGN UP FOR A GYM MEMBERSHIP

If it's January, then you might have to fight the crowds of people, fresh and full of enthusiasm after listing their resolutions for the New Year. But if you're out of shape, the best time to get started is right now with whatever you've got available. Take the time to get your new membership at a gym that is convenient to get to and makes you feel comfortable to be in. Get a fitness book with a few plans you can use to tailor your workout, or spend the extra cheddar on getting a personal trainer, who should also be convenient to go to and makes you feel comfortable to be around. Focus on regular visits for a span of three to four months, and hopefully by that time, you will find yourself hooked on the gym experience.

11

PUT ON A SMILE AND HUG IT OUT WITH SOMEONE

Putting a smile on your face will not only put an instant boost in your mood, but your smile will also brighten someone else's day. And studies show the simple act of hugging induces a positive chemical response in the body by increasing oxytocin (known as the hormone of love) and reducing cortisol levels (linked to chronic stress and can weaken the activity of the immune system). A 20-second hug can go a long way towards lowering your stress.

12

KNOCK OUT A SIXTY SECOND WORKOUT

Getting in a quick minute of exercise is a great way to gain a quick burst of energy when needed. Your goal is to get your blood just slightly pumping. Don't do anything that will work up a heavy sweat or will turn out to be too strenuous. Keep your mini workout along the lines of doing a few jumping jacks, a couple of push-ups or maybe even a set of lunges.

13

TIDY UP A NEGLECTED SPOT

Toss a few old things that are taking up space in the back of a closet. Clear all the toys--juvenile and adult--from under all the beds. Thoroughly vacuum or sweep under all of your furniture. Dust off the top of your refrigerator. It might not be a spot that will catch the attention of a regular house guest, but it will make you feel a lot better to know just how clean some of the commonly unseen areas of your house are.

14

CONNECT MORE PEOPLE TO MORE PEOPLE

Do you know a few people who could greatly benefit from making a connection with a few of your associate contacts? Start working on making more introductions on behalf of others. Be sure to refer some of your friends and favorite clients to other businesses people in your circle that offer products or services they may also need.

15

EAT AN EASIER BREAKFAST

Making sure you start off your day satisfied and not starved is the main purpose of getting a well-balanced breakfast every morning. But if your schedule or lifestyle does not translate well to a slow, sit down morning meal, a quick spread of peanut butter on a piece of toast or a bagel should always fit into your schedule. Even better, a pot of hard boiled eggs prepared on a Sunday night will sit well in the fridge all week for an easy grab-and-go breakfast. Stash a box of instant oatmeal packets in the back of a desk drawer at work for those mornings when you make it to the road without a pit stop in the kitchen before your commute. And if your break room vending machine turns into your only option, reaching for a breakfast bar or even a toaster pastry is still marginally better than a standard candy bar.

16

GET AROUND
TO THAT
TO THAT
FOLLOW UP

Those quick moments between appointments could be set aside for playing games on your smartphone, but should also allow for a great chance to increase your overall productivity. Those moments are perfect for reaching out and making contact with that person who you have neglected to contact. You probably only have a short available window to talk, so if you are making a phone call, you will be forced to keep the conversation short. This will keep you from getting sucked into a long, drawn out discussion--whether it is a safety net as a person who enjoys these conversations or an excuse for those who hate them. You can also use the opportunity to send out some quick emails to potential clients you have met, asking them, 'How can I help you?'

17

GET SOME STRESS RELIEF

Continued stress will do serious damage to your body, mind, and spirit. The easiest way to relieve stress from your body is just to give your body rest, but finding the time to do this has become more difficult in our new reality. But you can make it work. If you cannot find time in your schedule for a full body massage, you can always find 60 seconds to give yourself a personal neck massage, slowly stretch and shrug your shoulders, or just take a slow and deep breath. Skip a TV sitcom and unwind with a 30 minute soak in the tub. Feel free to set up the optional candles, aromatherapy, bath soaps, and a chilled glass of wine.

18

CALL YOUR MOM (AND DAD) AND TELL HER YOU LOVE HER (AND HIM)

It is almost impossible to call your parents too often. Almost. If you happen to have parents that are taking full advantage of their empty nester status by staying away from home and keeping the nest empty, then you may interrupt a session of your parents doing something that seems crazy that you may not want to think about. But chances are, your mother is telling you that you should be calling home more. Here, it really is impossible to call home too much in her eyes, even if you are calling daily. You are probably not going to start calling daily, but plan a regular time weekly to make contact. And since your parents are probably pretty hip with their smartphones, tablets, and laptops, try a few sessions of video chat. Don't be surprised if they start to get a little 'too busy' to accept those calls. Laugh it off and don't miss your scheduled time next week.

19

BE BETTER TO YOUR OTHER MOTHER (EARTH)

Crying Native Americans, animated bears, and people in owl costumes had a hard time in the past in spreading the message of being friendlier to this planet we call our home. Now, caring for the environment is big business, but it does not mean it is always efficiently done. You do not half to walk away from civilization to protect the planet. Start by refilling a non-disposable water bottle, always carry reusable canvas bags to the grocery store, and if your city has a recycling program, participate! Composting and driving electric cars is great, but pretty drastic for most people. Just a few simple changes in your lifestyle will add a dramatically positive effect on the world around you.

20

REVIEW AND REVISE YOUR SCHEDULE

A few spare minutes can allow you the chance to review your schedule to ensure it still meets your personal needs. Making a habit of doing periodic reviews of your schedule for regular updates is even better and can still take as little as a few minutes. You do not have a personal schedule that you consistently follow? These spare minutes are a good time to get started on one.

Remember, you should not fear becoming a slave to the schedule you create. Focus on the newfound freedom you will receive from uncertainty and unscheduled interruptions.

21

QUIT FORGETTING YOUR PASSWORDS

Make a list of all of your computer passwords and store that list in a safe place. This allows you access to your passwords should you forget one--or a few--and allow friends and loved one's access to your passwords and in turn your accounts in case of an emergency. It is also a good time to upgrade your password system. Stop reusing the same password, and avoid using simple and easy to crack passwords. The top five most used passwords in 2012 were, in reverse order: 5) qwerty, 4) abc123, 3) 12345678, 2) 123456, and 1) password. If any of these passwords look a little too familiar, change them immediately.

22

DROP AND GIVE YOURSELF 20

Much like the earlier suggestion of a 60-second workout, but this time, with the intensity of having a personal drill instructor barking orders your way. Give yourself 60 seconds to do as many pushups or crunches as you can. The first time you attempt these 60 second sprint exercises, it may seem like a struggle. It may make your quick minute seem much, much longer than a mere 60 seconds. But the more times you do it, the more you will be able to do, and longer. It will not take long before you will be able to feel, and then see, a difference.

23

GET A LITTLE FRUITY & NUTTY

Cut up a piece of fresh fruit and put it in an airtight storage container. This ensures that you have readily available healthy snack choices as a first option. Stock up on dried fruit and nuts, placing proper portion amounts into sandwich bags for the same result. If you are honestly short on prep time, buy plenty of protein and granola bars to stash away to stave off hunger pangs. Just be sure to keep an eye on the calorie count of the store bought bars. If you find you have a little extra time on your hand, do an internet search for a good recipe and make your own from scratch.

24

CALL FOR A 60-SECOND SCRUBBING

Have a package of pre-treated cleaning cloths or some old rags readily available for those quick moments that occur when you notice a smudge that needs wiping. Light switches and door handles are obvious spots since people are always touching them. But do not forget about mirrors and glass doors, magnets for finger prints and other greasy spots.

25

HANDWRITE A PERSONAL NOTE

Yes, you could send a text message and ensure instant delivery, but few actions and activities show just how much you care about a relationship, both business and personal, than passing a note written by one's own hand. You do not even have to go out and buy fancy stationery, as in most cases a few words jotted on a sticky note will do the trick.

26

CONNECT WITH SOCIAL MEDIA FOLLOWERS

You have spent a lot of time finding friends, fans, and followers using social media sites like Twitter and Facebook. But if you are not spending much time communicating with your 'peeps,' why should they continue to be your peeps? Send out regular updates of substance to all that follow you. Don't tell them you are having a sandwich for lunch. Tell them you are having a special lunch with a mentor, a beloved friend, or a rock star, and what it means to you. Send out words of encouragement to your followers, even if it is a cheesy clichéd motivational quote. Reach out to folks you have not chatted with in a while and ask them how they are doing, and be interested in their response. Don't fool yourself into believing that you truly have as many 'friends' as your profile may list, but be sure you have some sort of influence over each and every person who has desired to follow you and your message, and respect that platform.

27

SHOW SOME PRIDE IN YOUR KIDS

As the father of a once former surly teenager, I know how it feels to search for positive things to say about your child when the child is growing out of the practice of doing positive things. As a former surly teenager, I know how good it felt for my parents to say positive things about me when I fell out of the habit of doing positive things. Children are not a possession. They are a precious gift, even when they are determined to be otherwise. Even if your child is extraordinarily special, they don't always know how you feel about them unless you speak the words. So tell your children just how proud you are of them. Then tell the world just how proud you are of your children. Then tell your children about how you just told the world how proud you are of them. Finding points of favor to promote is easier than you think.

28

CHECK YOUR TIRE PRESSURE

A common phrase you will hear from your mechanic is 'pay me now or pay me later,' referring to the cost of maintenance versus the cost of repairs. A little vigilance on your point will keep you one step ahead of your maintenance schedule, and totally prepared for any real emergencies. Keeping an eye on the pressure in your tires will ensure your car gets efficient gas mileage all year, and ride safer on the roads in winter conditions. Staying mindful of the mileage between oil changes will keep you on schedule for regular maintenance. And regular runs through the car wash or stops for detailing will make you look and feel better in your ride.

29

GIVE YOUR EYES A BREAK

The glare coming from your computer is doing damage to your eyes. It may be subtle, but it is doing more damage than you may think. Schedule some time every hour to look away from your computer. Do not just call it a break, blink twice, and go back to tapping at the keyboard. Have a non-LCD glaring activity awaiting your scheduled break. Look out the window, file some paperwork, read a physical book (with page made out of paper), maybe even leave your desk for a walk outside. Whatever you do, just make sure it is not an activity that leads you from staring at one screen to staring at a totally different screen.

30

STOP WAITING
TO EXHALE

Stopping to do breathing exercises on a regular basis will help you maintain a balanced level of stress, even on completely chaotic days. A standard breathing exercise known as 'balanced breathing' is a good place to start. Inhale for a count of four through the nose, and then exhale for a count of four, again through the nose. This adds a natural resistance to the act of breathing and forces you to keep breaths balanced. As your skill in this exercise increases, you can increase your breath counts to as much as ten, or add in the abdominal breathing technique, placing one hand on your chest and the other hand on your stomach to ensure you are breathing through your diaphragm.

31

ENGAGE THE POWER OF VISUALIZATION

While many still mock the 'spell' that the book *The Secret* cast over many of its readers, the fact remains that there is actual merit to the power of attraction. The things you focus on the most tend to be the things that affect you most in life. So if you have a few spare minutes, take some time to close your eyes and play some positive images into your mind. Making this a daily habit will go a long way to battling the negativity of the outside world and the fear you battle in the world inside your own head.

32

TAKE IT TO A HIGHER POWER

Even if you are an atheist or agnostic, I believe one would be foolish to believe that the universe is comprised of completely random events. Your destiny, or whatever you wish to call it, is determined by the events and decisions you make minute by minute throughout your day. In this book about what to do when you find spare minutes in your day, I suggest taking a moment to pray about your decisions to whatever deity you happen to choose, and saying you do not follow a religion does not get you off the hook. Call it a reflection or evaluation of your choices if you must. The world is bigger than the person you are, and we all have some effect in each other's lives, as minor as it may seem at the moment. So live outside of the moment, and seek a greater understanding, or Higher Power, to guide you.

33

DRINK A GLASS OF WATER

The debate continues to rage on whether the average person needs 8 glasses of water a day. Some need 8, some need more or less, and some have a problem with what is considered 'average.' But we all need water, and except for extremely rare cases, a little more water will not hurt you (other than needing to take more trips to the bathroom through the day). Try starting out your morning by drinking a glass water, in whatever size you like, as soon as you get out of bed. Then, as you go through your day, grab some water to sip or chug between (or instead of) hits of coffee, tea, and soda. It should help stave off hunger, add moisture to your skin, and relieve boredom.

ABOUT THE AUTHOR

J Cleveland Payne is a reluctant 'jack of all trades,' and a surprising master of many of them. A United States Air Force veteran, 20-year broadcasting professional and longtime student of leadership and personal development, Payne works daily with companies and individuals to help them evaluate their current states of reality and create plans of action to help them move forward to a better one. He would rather be yakking on the radio as a talk show host, but until that can become a full-time gig, he is glad to have the chance every day to assist a variety of people as they work on their progress.

You can read more words from Payne by visiting his website, jclevelandpayne.net and you can email him your own words at mailbox@jclevelandpayne.net.

ASK YOURSELF THIS
A DAILY QUOTES & QUESTIONS
WORKBOOK FEATURING 366 THOUGHTS TO
JUMP START YOUR MIND EVERYDAY

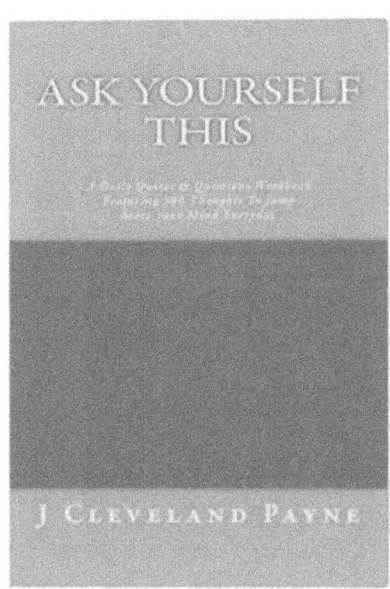

Ask Yourself This is a simple workbook with a simple purpose: providing you a daily quote and a daily question inspired by that quote. Every page is dates (even February 29th) and provides adequate writing space that enables you to use the book as a personal journal that you can easily reference back to in the future. Day by day and question by question, you will get a mental boost that will lead you to a clearer and more open view of the world around you, along with the world inside you.

**AVAILABLE IN PAPERBACK AT
AMAZOM.COM**

GET ALL THE BOOKS IN THE #MONDAYMESSAGE SERIES

WELCOME TO YOUR MONDAY

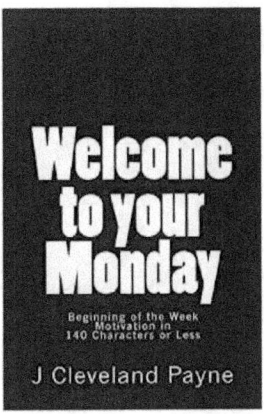

The Original Amazon Kindle
Best Seller That Puts A
Year's Worth Of Quick
Motivational Messages In
The Palm Of Your Hand

Visit Amazon.com
and search for
'Welcome to your Monday'

WELCOME TO MORE MONDAYS

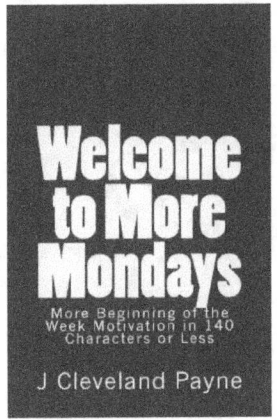

The Series Continues
With Another Full Year's
Worth Of Quick
Motivational Messages To Kee
Your Spirits Up

Visit Amazon.com
and search for
'Welcome to More Monday'

Your Problem Is That You Need Is A Dynamic Speaker For Your Group Or Event...

Your Problem Is Solved By Making Contact With J Cleveland Payne...

Payne Has Created Speeches And Programs That Cover A Variety Of Topics, To Include **Leadership, Followership, Planning & Continuity, Motivation, Storytelling, Broadcast Media Preparation, Social Media Mastery, Keeping A Positive Mindset While Living In A Negative World.**

Make Contact By Visiting jclevelandpayne.net Or Calling (501) 240-9670